CANCER CAREGIVER'S HANDBOOK

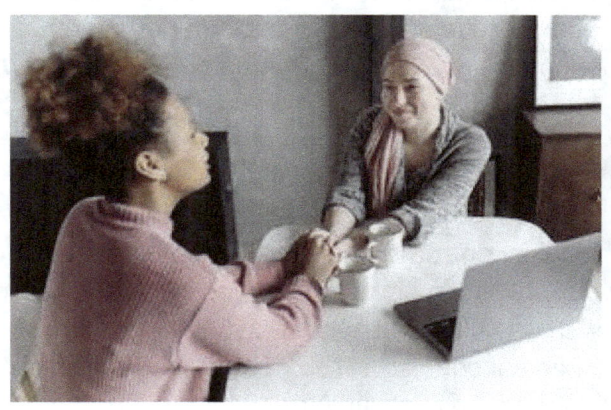

A Guide to Supporting Your Loved One Through Treatment and Recovery

DENI DERA

APPRECIATION

Writing a book is a journey filled with challenges and discoveries, and it's a journey I didn't take alone. I want to express my deepest appreciation to all those who contributed to the creation of this work..

To my editor, whose keen eye and insightful suggestions polished this manuscript into its final form. Your dedication to excellence is truly commendable. To the readers, who have chosen to embark on this journey with me, I am deeply grateful for your time and trust. It is my hope that the words within these pages bring you value, inspiration, and perhaps even a new perspective.

And lastly, to the countless individuals who face the challenges of cancer with courage and resilience every day, you are the true heroes. It is for you that this book was written, and it is with the utmost respect and admiration that I dedicate it to all those affected by cancer.

DEDICATION

To all those touched by the profound
journey of cancer – the fighters, the
survivors, the caregivers, and the
champions of hope. Your strength and
resilience inspire this work.

TABLE OF CONTENT

APPRECIATION   1

DEDICATION   3

TABLE OF CONTENT   4

INTRODUCTION   6

Who's A Caregiver   9

Who Is a Cancer Caregiver Not?   12

IMPORTANCE OF SUPPORT FOR THE
PATIENT AND CAREGIVER   14

Note to the Patient: 15

Note to the Caregiver: 16

UNDERSTANDING CANCER   18

What exactly is cancer?   19

Risk Factors and Causes: 19

Types and stages of cancer   22

Cancer Types: 22

Cancer Stages: 24

Treatment options and their side effects   27

Emotional impact of cancer on patients and
caregivers   31

Cancer Patients' Emotional Impact: 32

Caregivers' Emotional Impact: 33

PREPARING FOR TREATMENT   36

Planning for hospital stays   36

Making treatment decisions   41

Support resources for patients and caregivers 45

Financial considerations related to cancer treatment 50

PROVIDING EMOTIONAL SUPPORT 55

- Managing caregiver burnout 59

ASSISTING WITH DAILY LIVING 63

Managing medications and treatments 67

Nutritional support and meal planning 73

When Patients Refuses Meals Or HealthCare Instructions 78

MANAGING SIDE EFFECTS 84

Navigating Common Side Effects: 85

Working with the Healthcare Team to Manage Symptoms: 86

Adapting to Changes in the Patient's Health: 87

COPING WITH TREATMENT CHANGES AND TRANSITIONS 90

End-of-treatment and survivorship resources 95

END-OF-LIFE CARE 101

CONCLUSION 108

Resources for Ongoing Assistance 109

Credits and acknowledgements 111

Appendix 113

List of resources for patients and caregivers 113

MEDICATION TRACKERS 117

INTRODUCTION

Cancer isn't simply a diagnosis for the person who receives it; it's also a diagnosis for their whole family, circle of friends, and community. In the face of such a terrible foe, the responsibility of a caretaker assumes extraordinary importance.

This is the "Cancer Caregiver's Handbook: A Guide to Supporting Your Loved One Through Treatment and Recovery." This book is a source of empowerment and direction for people who find themselves in the role of caregiver, standing shoulder to shoulder with a loved one confronting cancer.

Caring for others is hard for the faint of heart; it needs resilience, compassion, and unflinching devotion. It's a journey that requires you to be a rock of strength while negotiating the difficult terrain of emotions, medical decisions, and day-to-day problems.

The goal of this manual is simple: to offer you with the information, skills, and support you need to be the greatest caregiver possible. Practical guidance, professional insights, and poignant anecdotes from others who have traveled this route before you may be found inside these pages. This book is intended to help you understand, support, and encourage the person you care about, whether you are a family member, a friend, a partner, or a neighbor.

We'll go through the essentials of caring, from the emotional toll it might take to the practicalities of scheduling appointments and taking prescriptions. You'll learn how to communicate effectively, deal with your own emotions, and seek help when necessary. We'll dig into the complexities of cancer treatment and recovery, deciphering medical jargon and equipping you to be an advocate for a loved one.

This guidebook, however, is more than simply a practical guide; it is a monument to the human spirit's strength and the power of compassion. It serves as a reminder that even in the darkest of circumstances, there is hope and healing.

Know that you are not alone as you begin on this road of caring. Countless others have traveled this route before you, and they are now standing with you, providing their wisdom and support. Your love and attention make an incalculable impact in the life of your loved one.

So, let us go on this voyage together. Allow the "Cancer Caregiver's Handbook" to be your constant companion as you negotiate the hurdles, provide consolation, and become a beacon of hope on the path to healing.

With compassion and tenacity,

Who's A Caregiver

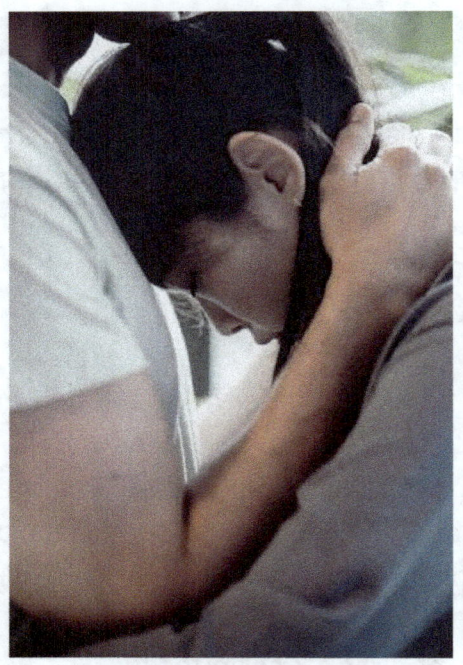

A cancer caregiver is someone who gives physical, emotional, and frequently logistical assistance to someone who has been diagnosed with cancer. Caregivers play an important part in the cancer journey, providing care and aid to their loved ones as they face the obstacles that illness entails.

A cancer caregiver's duties might vary greatly and may include:

1. **Emotional Support:** Being a listening ear, offering consolation, and being a source of emotional strength for the cancer patient.

2. **Assistance with Daily Activities:** Assisting with duties such as washing, clothing, meal preparation, and medication administration, especially if the person with cancer is suffering physical restrictions due to treatment or sickness.

3. **Accompanying to Medical visits:** Attending doctor's visits and treatments, taking notes, and asking questions on behalf of the cancer patient.

4. **Advocacy:** Acting as an advocate to ensure the person with cancer obtains the best possible treatment, including collaborating with medical experts, insurance providers, and support services.

5. **Logistical Support:** Handling practical things such as transportation to and from

medical appointments, managing funds, and arranging healthcare-related paperwork.

6. **Providing Information:** Researching and sharing information regarding the cancer diagnosis, treatment choices, and potential side effects to assist the cancer patient in making educated decisions.

7. **Providing Companionship:** Spending meaningful time with the cancer patient, participating in talks, hobbies, or pastimes to lessen feelings of isolation and loneliness.

8. **Respite Care:** Arranging for temporary relief to reduce caregiver fatigue. This may entail obtaining assistance from other family members, friends, or respite care agencies.
Cancer caring may be emotionally and physically taxing, and carers frequently encounter their own set of problems and anxieties. They do, however, play an important part in the well-being and rehabilitation of the cancer patient, providing critical support during a tough period.

Cancer caregivers must prioritize self-care, seek support from support groups or specialists when required, and speak freely with the person they are caring for to ensure that both parties receive the assistance and emotional support they deserve.

Who Is a Cancer Caregiver Not?

A cancer caregiver is not a medical practitioner or healthcare provider who is responsible for diagnosing, treating, or actively managing the medical aspects of cancer. A cancer caregiver is a caring somebody, generally a family member, friend, or loved one, who provides aid, emotional support, and practical assistance to someone diagnosed with cancer.

A cancer carer is not:

1. **A Medical Expert:** A cancer caregiver is not a doctor, nurse, or healthcare professional. They do not make medical

decisions or give medical care to the cancer patient.

2. **A Substitute for Professional Care:** While carers play an important role in providing assistance, they are not a replacement for the knowledge and care offered by qualified medical professionals. Healthcare professionals make medical choices and administer treatments.

3. **A Cure Provider:** Caregivers are not responsible for discovering a cure for cancer. Their duty is to provide comfort, friendship, and aid to the cancer patient throughout their journey.

4. **A Replacement for Self-Care:** Caregivers must prioritize self-care to minimize caregiver burnout and preserve their own physical and mental well-being. They are not asked to compromise their own health for the sake of caregiving.

5. **A Medical Decision-Maker:** While caregivers may provide input and support in decision-making processes, the person

diagnosed with cancer and their healthcare team make the final decisions regarding medical treatments and care plans.

6. A **Financial Advisor:** While caregivers may assist with practical concerns such as managing funds and insurance, they are not financial experts and are not responsible for making financial decisions for the person with cancer.

In short, a cancer caregiver is a sympathetic and helpful somebody who aids and soothes someone dealing with cancer, but they do not assume the medical or professional obligations connected with diagnosing or treating the disease. A caregiver's job is to provide emotional, physical, and practical assistance at a difficult time.

IMPORTANCE OF SUPPORT FOR THE PATIENT AND CAREGIVER

During the difficult road of cancer diagnosis, treatment, and recovery, it is critical to have support for both the patient and the caregiver. This is why:

Note to the Patient:

1. Emotional Health: Fear, worry, and uncertainty often accompany a cancer diagnosis. Caregivers, family, and friends provide emotional support to patients, decreasing stress and increasing mental well-being.

2. Encouragement: Knowing that someone cares passionately about their well-being can motivate patients to stick to treatment regimens, retain a good perspective, and persevere in the face of adversity.

3. Assistance in Practice: Patients frequently encounter physical issues as a result of their therapies, making daily chores difficult. Caregivers assist with everyday duties such as cooking, transportation, and medication administration.

Advocacy: Medical information and decisions may be overwhelming for patients. Caregivers can act as advocates, assisting patients in understanding treatment options, communicating with healthcare experts, and making educated decisions.

5. Lower Isolation: Cancer may be isolating, causing sufferers to withdraw from social situations. Support from caregivers and loved ones guarantees that they do not feel isolated and detached from the rest of the world.

Note to the Caregiver:

1. Decreased Burnout: Caring for others may be physically and emotionally draining. The presence of a support system minimizes caregiver burnout, allowing them to deliver better care to the patient.

2. Emotional Release: Caregivers feel a variety of emotions, including worry, despair, and frustration. It may be therapeutic and emotionally soothing to have someone to talk to and express their thoughts with.

3. Assistance in Practice: Caregivers, like patients, may require assistance from friends

and family to manage their obligations and ensure they have time to relax and care for themselves.

4. Information and Education: Caregivers can have access to resources, information, and education about the condition, treatment choices, and how to offer best care through support networks.

Validation: Caregivers may have doubts about their abilities or judgments from time to time. Others' support validates their efforts and underlines the critical role they play in the patient's life.

In essence, the journey through cancer is one that the patient and caregiver share. Friends, family, and the healthcare team's support deepens this relationship, allowing both the patient and caregiver to face the difficulties and uncertainties of cancer with resilience, optimism, and enhanced quality of life. It emphasizes the idea that in the face of misfortune, the strength of a caring community can make all the difference.

UNDERSTANDING CANCER

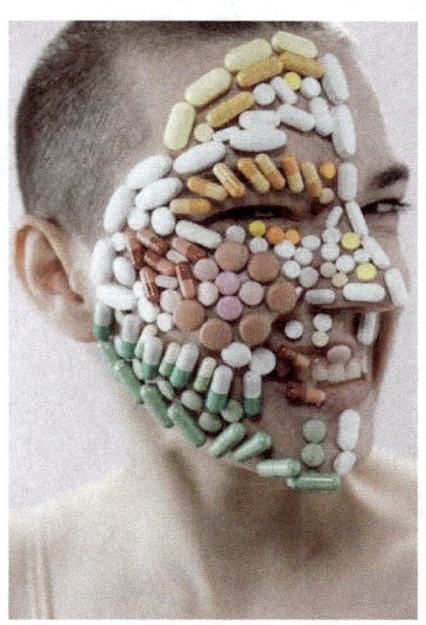

Cancer, in all of its manifestations, is one of the most difficult and complicated diseases known to man. Its frequency, diversity, and often catastrophic impact on people and families have prompted much investigation and study. Understanding cancer entails delving into the complicated network of biology, genetics, lifestyle variables, and medicinal advances that characterize the illness.

What exactly is cancer?

Cancer is, at its core, a collection of illnesses characterized by the uncontrolled development and spread of aberrant cells. Normal cells in the body grow, divide, and die in a predictable way. Cancer cells, on the other hand, deviate from this tightly controlled mechanism, resulting in the creation of tumors or the invasion of neighboring tissues and organs.

Risk Factors and Causes:

Cancer is caused by a confluence of hereditary, environmental, and lifestyle factors. Exposure to carcinogens (cancer-causing chemicals), a family history of cancer, certain illnesses, and unhealthy behaviors such as smoking, poor nutrition, and lack of physical activity are all established risk factors.

Early detection and prevention:

While not all malignancies can be avoided, there are steps people may do to minimize their risk. Maintaining a good diet, staying physically active, limiting alcohol use, and avoiding tobacco products are all lifestyle choices that can dramatically reduce the chance of acquiring cancer.

Additionally, early detection is crucial. Cancer screenings and self-examinations on a regular basis can aid in the detection of cancer in its early, more curable stages. Screening procedures include mammograms, Pap smears, colonoscopies, and prostate-specific antigen (PSA) testing.

Treatment Advances:

Cancer therapy has come a long way in recent years. Surgery, radiation therapy, chemotherapy, immunotherapy, targeted treatments, and precision medicine are common treatment options. Treatment options are determined by criteria such as cancer kind, stage, and specific patient characteristics.

Assistance and Research:

Support networks, such as caregivers, healthcare professionals, and cancer support organizations, are critical in assisting people and families in coping with the physical and emotional problems of cancer. Cancer research continues to grow, leading to the development of novel medicines and measures for prevention and early detection.

Understanding cancer is a never-ending process distinguished by scientific advancements, medical breakthroughs, and the tenacity of individuals affected. While cancer remains a powerful foe, the combined efforts of researchers, healthcare professionals, patients, and caregivers provide hope for better therapies, better outcomes, and, eventually, a future where cancer is preventable and cured.

Types and stages of cancer

Cancer is, without a doubt, a complicated illness with different forms and stages. I'll go through some of the most prevalent cancer kinds and stages here:

Cancer Types:

Carcinoma: Carcinomas are tumors that arise in the epithelial cells that cover the organ, skin, and gland surfaces. The most prevalent kinds are as follows:

- Adenocarcinoma: Forms in glandular tissue and is commonly detected in organs such as the breast, prostate, and colon.
- Squamous Cell Carcinoma: This type of cancer develops in the squamous cells that line the skin and organs including the lungs and esophagus.

Sarcoma: Sarcomas develop in connective tissues such as bones, muscles, and cartilage.

Leukemia: Leukemia affects the blood and bone marrow, disrupting normal blood cell formation. Acute lymphoblastic leukemia (ALL) and chronic myeloid leukemia (CML) are two kinds of leukemia.

Lymphoma: Lymphomas start in the lymphatic system, particularly in the lymph nodes and lymphatic tissues. Hodgkin lymphoma and non-Hodgkin lymphoma are the two primary forms.

Melanoma: Melanoma is a kind of skin cancer that originates in melanocytes, the pigment-producing cells of the skin. If not discovered early, it can be quite aggressive.

Cancers of the Central Nervous System (CNS): These tumors manifest themselves in the brain and spinal cord. Examples include gliomas, meningiomas, and medulloblastomas.

Carcinoid Tumors: The gastrointestinal system, particularly the small intestine and appendix, is the most common location for these tumors.

Cancer Stages:

Cancer staging is a classification system that describes the amount and severity of cancer in the body. The TNM system is the most often used staging system:

1. **T (Tumor):** This reflects the main tumor's size and extent. T0 indicates that there is no indication of a tumor, but higher numbers (e.g., T1, T2, T3, T4) show the size and extent of the tumor.

2. **N (Nodes):** Indicates whether or not the malignancy has spread to surrounding lymph nodes. N0 indicates that there are no lymph nodes involved, but N1, N2, and N3 show the degree of lymph node involvement.

3. **M (Metastasis):** M0 shows that cancer has not moved to other organs, but M1 indicates that cancer has disseminated to distant places.

Cancer is staged after the TNM categories are determined:

- **Stage 0 (on-site):** Cancer is restricted to the spot where it originated and has not invaded or spread to surrounding tissues. Surgery or targeted therapy may be used as treatment alternatives.

- **First Stage:** Cancer is confined and very tiny at this stage. It has not yet infiltrated neighboring tissues or organs. Surgical removal of the tumor is a common treatment option.

- **Tier II:** At this stage, the cancer may be more advanced and may have spread to surrounding tissues or lymph nodes. The spread decides whether it is classified as Stage IIA or IIB. Surgery, radiation therapy, and chemotherapy are all options for treatment.

- **Tier III:** Cancer has usually increased in size and spread to surrounding lymph nodes or tissues. Stage IIIA, IIIB, and IIIC are subgroups based on the amount of local invasion and lymph node involvement. Surgery, radiation, and chemotherapy are frequently used in treatment.

- **Tier IV:** Cancer has spread to distant organs or tissues at this stage. It is frequently thought to be metastatic. Treatment seeks to manage symptoms, restrict cancer spread, and improve the patient's quality of life. Targeted treatments, immunotherapies, and palliative care may be used

Staging aids in treatment decisions, determining prognosis, and determining the amount of cancer's spread throughout the body. The precise staging system may differ based on the kind of cancer, however the TNM system serves as a broad framework. Early identification and precise staging are critical for designing successful treatment options and improving cancer patient outcomes.

Cancer stage is important in determining prognosis and therapy choices. In general, earlier-stage malignancies have better prognosis and a higher possibility of cure. Even in late stages, there are therapy choices that can help manage the disease, relieve symptoms, and extend lives.

It's crucial to note that not all cancers fit neatly into the TNM staging method, since some have their own set of criteria. Furthermore, cancer staging is always changing as our understanding of the illness and treatment choices improves. It is critical to contact with healthcare specialists and oncologists that specialize in the specific cancer diagnosis for accurate and up-to-date information on cancer kinds and their unique staging.

Let us proceed with additional information about cancer phases and their implications:

Treatment options and their side effects

Cancer therapy options have substantially improved throughout the years, providing a variety of techniques to tackle the illness. These therapies, however, can have adverse effects that vary based on the type of therapy utilized and particular patient variables. Here's a rundown of some of the most prevalent cancer treatments and their possible adverse effects:

1. **Surgery:**
<u>Treatment</u>: Surgical removal of malignant tumors or tissue.

- Side Effects: Pain, swelling, bleeding, infection at the surgical site, scars, and functional changes (e.g., loss of mobility or organ function) depending on the location of the surgery.

2. **Radiation Therapy:**
<u>Treatment</u>: Radiation beams with high intensity target and destroy cancer cells.

- adverse Effects: Skin irritation, weariness, nausea, and treatment-specific adverse effects (e.g., hair loss, trouble swallowing, bowel or bladder problems). The majority of adverse effects are quite transient.

3. **Chemotherapy:**

Treatment: Medications target cancer cells that are rapidly developing throughout the body.

   - Side Effects: Nausea, vomiting, hair loss, exhaustion, reduced blood cell counts (increased risk of infections and bleeding), appetite changes, and susceptibility to infections.

4. **Immunotherapy:**

   Treatment: Increases the body's immune system's ability to identify and destroy cancer cells.

   - Adverse Reactions: Immune-related symptoms include tiredness, rash, fever, diarrhea, and, in rare cases, severe autoimmune responses involving several organs. Immunotherapy has fewer negative effects than standard chemotherapy.

5. **Targeted Therapy:**

   Treatment: Specific molecules involved in cancer development and progression are targeted.

   - Adverse Reactions: Skin rashes, diarrhea, high blood pressure, and liver issues are frequent adverse effects that might vary based on the precise targeted treatment employed.

6. **Hormone Therapy:**
<u>Treatment</u>: Used to slow or halt cancer growth in hormone-sensitive cancers by interfering with the body's hormonal signals.
- Side Effects: Menopausal symptoms (such as hot flashes and mood swings), exhaustion, weight gain, and bone density abnormalities.

7. **Stem Cell Transplant:**
<u>Treatment</u>: Replaces damaged or destroyed bone marrow with healthy stem cells, commonly utilized in the treatment of blood-related malignancies.
- Adverse Reactions: Weakening of the immune system, higher risk of infections, weariness, nausea, and, in certain circumstances, graft-versus-host disease (in which donor cells attack the tissues of the recipient).

8. **Palliative Care:**
<u>Treatment</u>: Emphasizes symptom management, pain alleviation, and increasing

the patient's quality of life, especially in advanced cancer patients.

- negative Effects: There are few negative effects, however it does not treat the cancer and is just used to offer comfort and support.

It is crucial to note that the adverse effects of cancer therapy might vary greatly between individuals. To successfully control side effects, healthcare personnel continuously monitor patients and modify treatment strategies. Furthermore, innovations in cancer care continue to result in medicines with fewer and milder side effects, improving both treatment efficacy and patient comfort.

Patients are advised to discuss potential side effects, concerns, and coping methods with their healthcare providers in order to make educated treatment decisions and successfully manage side effects.

Emotional impact of cancer on patients and caregivers

Cancer has a significant and complicated emotional impact on both patients and caregivers. Coping with a cancer diagnosis and treatment is an emotional rollercoaster that is typically packed with a wide variety of powerful emotions. The following is an examination of the emotional impact on both groups:

Cancer Patients' Emotional Impact:

1. **Disbelief and Shock:** After getting a cancer diagnosis, many people suffer shock and disbelief. Denial may act as a protective strategy in the face of overwhelming news.

2. **Anxiety and Fear:** Fear of the unknown, worries about the future, and worry about treatment success and potential repercussions are all prevalent feelings.

3. **Depression and Grief:** Cancer patients may be saddened by the physical and mental changes they undergo throughout treatment, as well as the loss of their pre-diagnosis lives.

4. **Frustration and Anger:** Cancer can induce annoyance and rage because of the disturbance it causes in a person's life. This might be aimed against the sickness, healthcare providers, or even family members.

5. **Loneliness and isolation:** Because of the physical and emotional toll of cancer, patients may feel alone. In addition, they may retreat from social activities and relationships.

6. **Depression:** Clinical depression is widespread among cancer patients as they cope with the disease's emotional toll and life-altering consequences.

7. **Optimism and Resilience:** Despite the difficulties, many patients discover inner strength and resilience, typically motivated by optimism and desire to beat the disease.

Caregivers' Emotional Impact:

1. **Anxiety and Fear:** Caregivers frequently share the patient's concerns about the

diagnosis, treatment outcomes, and the future.

2. **Guilt and Impotence:** Caregivers may feel guilty, as if they aren't doing enough, or as if they contributed to the disease. They may also feel powerless in the face of the patient's pain.

3. **Stress and Fatigue:** Caring for a cancer patient may be both physically and emotionally taxing. Caregivers who mix caring obligations with their own life may endure stress, weariness, and burnout.

4. **Depression and Grief:** Caregivers may experience sadness and loss as a result of witnessing a loved one's suffering and changes in health.

5. **Dispute and Relationship Stress:** Caregiving stress may strain relationships. Caregivers may get angry or resentful, and family disputes may emerge.

6. **Isolation:** Due to the duties of caring, caregivers may withdraw themselves from social activities or endure social isolation.

7. **Patience and Hope:** Despite the difficulties, many carers find hope in helping their loved ones and acquire a strong feeling of compassion and empathy.

It's crucial to remember that at different points of the cancer journey, both patients and caregivers may experience a combination of these emotions. Open and honest communication, seeking help from healthcare experts, therapists, support groups, and friends, and practicing self-care are all important ways for dealing with the emotional effect of cancer on both patients and caregivers.

PREPARING FOR TREATMENT

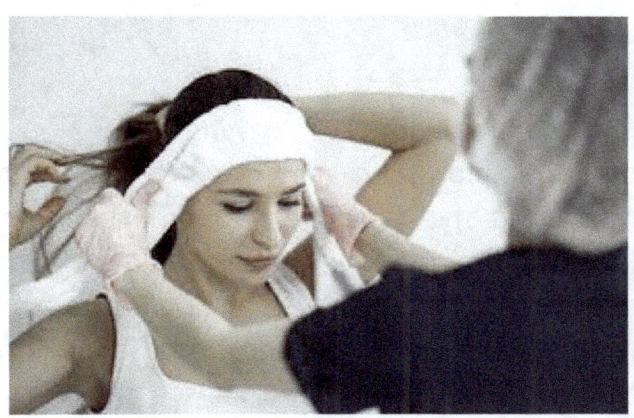

Cancer therapy preparation is a vital stage in the cancer process. It entails a number of critical procedures to ensure that both patients and caregivers are well-informed, psychologically and emotionally prepared, and physically prepared for the therapy ahead.

Planning for hospital stays

It is critical to plan ahead of time for hospital stays during cancer treatment to ensure a seamless and enjoyable experience. Hospitalization may be necessary for a variety of reasons, such as surgery, rigorous therapy, or complications. Here's a guide on preparing for hospital visits during cancer treatment:

1. **Communication:** Maintain open communication with your healthcare staff to understand the reason of your hospital stay and the projected length of your stay. Discuss your treatment strategy, anticipated adverse effects, and any preparations that are required.

2. **Essentials for Packing:** Make a hospital packing list, which should include personal hygiene supplies, comfortable clothing, slippers or non-slip socks, and any comfort items, such as a favorite blanket or pillow. Don't forget to bring important papers including identification, insurance cards, and medical records.

3. **Medication Management:** Make a list of all your current medications, including doses and regimens. Bring your drugs to the

hospital or offer this information to the medical staff.

4. **Advance Directives:** Review and update your advance directives, which should include a living will and healthcare proxy. Make certain that your preferred decision-maker is aware of your choices.

5. **Personal Belongings:** During your hospital stay, keep important goods and cash at home or with a trusted friend or family member to avoid loss or theft.

6. **Notify Loved Ones:** Inform relatives and friends about your anticipated hospital stay, its estimated duration, and how they may reach you while you are there.

7. **Childcare and Pet Care:** If required, arrange for childcare or pet care. Make sure your dependents are taken care of while you are in the hospital.

8. **Transportation:** Arrange for transportation to and from the hospital, whether by automobile, public transit, or ambulance.

Ascertain that you have contact information for dependable transportation choices.

9. **Caregivers' Accommodation:** If you will be accompanied by a caregiver, check about available caregiver lodgings near the hospital. Some institutions provide carers with accommodation or adjacent lodgings.

10. **Healthcare Proxy:** If you have a healthcare proxy, or someone who makes medical decisions on your behalf, make sure they are aware of your hospital stay and treatment choices.

11. **Financial Considerations:** Examine your insurance coverage and learn about the financial implications of your hospital stay. Contact your insurance provider to discuss coverage and any pre-authorizations that may be required.

12. **Support System:** Inform your support system about your hospital stay so that they can help with logistics like transportation, meal delivery, and emotional support.

Bring personal comfort items that create a sense of familiarity and relaxation, such as literature, music, or a tablet for amusement.

14. **Be Informed:** Be aware of your treatment plan, anticipated procedures, and any adverse effects. As required, ask your healthcare team questions and seek clarity.

15. **Emergency Contacts:** Share emergency contact information with your healthcare team and, if applicable, your caregiver.

16. **Health Record:** During your hospital stay, keep a diary or health record to track your symptoms, medications, and any concerns. Communication and decision-making can benefit from this.

17. **Adhere to Hospital procedures:** Observe hospital procedures regarding visiting hours, COVID-19 limits, and other safety precautions.

Remember that hospital stays during cancer treatment can be difficult, but careful planning can make the experience more bearable. Throughout your hospital stay, rely on your healthcare team and support network for direction and help, and don't be afraid to express any concerns or preferences to ensure you get the best treatment possible.

Making treatment decisions

Making treatment decisions in the context of cancer is one of the most important and difficult components of the trip. These decisions may include selecting from a variety of treatment alternatives, balancing possible advantages and risks, and taking into account personal beliefs and preferences. Here's a detailed guide to determining treatment options after being diagnosed with cancer:

1. **Obtain Information:** Begin by gathering as much information as possible regarding your cancer diagnosis. Learn about the kind, stage, and grade of your cancer, as well as the treatment options available. Your

healthcare team will be an invaluable resource.

2. **Seek views from experts:** Obtain views and consultations from cancer experts such as medical oncologists, surgeons, radiation oncologists, and others. Consider getting a second opinion to ensure you have a well-rounded view of your treatment choices.

3. **Know Your Treatment Options:** Educate yourself on the different treatment methods available, including as surgery, chemotherapy, radiation therapy, immunotherapy, targeted therapy, hormone therapy, and palliative care. Each sort of treatment has its own set of aims and potential adverse effects.

4. **Discuss Treatment Objectives:** Discuss your treatment objectives with your healthcare team in an open and honest manner. Is your goal to cure, control the disease, treat symptoms, or provide palliative care? Clarifying your objectives is critical for directing therapy selections.

5. **Get Second Opinions:** If you have any issues or concerns about your first treatment suggestions, get a second opinion. Different doctors' viewpoints and treatment choices may differ.

6. **Weigh dangers and advantages:** Identify the possible advantages and dangers of each treatment choice. Examine how each therapy may influence your quality of life, taking into account potential side effects and long-term repercussions.

7. **Examine Your Personal Values and Preferences**

- Consider your own personal values, priorities, and preferences. What are your therapy objectives? What are your thoughts on probable side effects and their influence on your everyday life?

8. **Involve Loved Ones:** Hold conversations with loved ones, family members, or carers. Their advice can give significant emotional support and assist you in making sound decisions.

9. **Pose Questions:** Don't be afraid to ask your healthcare staff questions and get clarity. Understanding the specifics of your treatment options is critical for making well-informed decisions.

10. **Seek assist:** Consider attending cancer support groups or consulting with a therapist to assist you manage the emotional implications of treatment decisions.

11 - **Take Your Time:** While prompt therapy is critical in cancer care, don't hurry into your decision. Take the time you need to acquire information, speak with experts, and carefully weigh your alternatives.

12. **Follow Your Instincts:** Finally, your treatment selections should be guided by your values, preferences, and degree of comfort. Trust your intuition and make decisions that seem good to you.

13. **Reassess and Adjust:** Cancer treatment strategies might change over time. Prepare to reassess your treatment choices as your

health evolves, and don't be afraid to revise your strategy if required.

14. **Maintain Open Communication:** Throughout your treatment, keep in touch with your healthcare team. Any concerns, adverse effects, or changes in your health should be communicated as soon as possible.

Making cancer treatment selections is a very personal experience. Each person's experience is unique, and the ideal treatment option may differ from one person to the next. Working closely with your healthcare team, using your support network, and prioritizing your well-being and values are critical when making decisions that affect your cancer treatment and overall quality of life.

Support resources for patients and caregivers

Cancer support resources are critical for giving aid, information, and emotional comfort to both cancer patients and carers throughout the cancer experience. These resources include a wide range of services and organizations devoted to meeting the medical, emotional, and practical needs of cancer patients. Here are some helpful resources:

1. **Healthcare Team:** Your healthcare team, which includes oncologists, nurses, and other medical experts, is your primary source of support. They give medical care, therapeutic advice, and information on how to manage adverse effects.

2. **Cancer Support Organizations:** Countless cancer-related organizations provide a plethora of information and support services. The American Cancer Society, CancerCare, and the Leukemia & Lymphoma Society are a few examples. These organizations provide instructional materials, support groups, and financial aid.

3. **Cancer Support Groups:** Cancer support groups bring together people who have had similar experiences. These organizations can give a sense of belonging, emotional support,

and practical help. They can be in-person or online, making them available to a wide spectrum of people.

4. **Caregiver Support Groups:** Specialized caregiver support groups are offered to assist carers in connecting with others who are facing similar issues. These organizations provide a forum for people to discuss their experiences, seek advice, and receive emotional support.

5. **Social Workers:** Hospitals and cancer centers frequently employ social workers who may help patients and caregivers navigate the healthcare system, link them with resources, and provide emotional support.

6. **Cancer Navigators:** Cancer navigators, also known as patient navigators, are specialists who are trained to help patients and carers navigate the complexity of cancer care. They provide individualized assistance and can assist in the coordination of appointments and resources.

7. **Palliative Care and Hospice Services:** Palliative care teams work to improve the quality of life for individuals suffering from severe illnesses such as cancer. Hospice care offers end-of-life care. Both services provide emotional and practical support.

8. **Online Resources:** Countless websites and online communities offer a plethora of information as well as places for interacting with people impacted by cancer. Websites such as Cancer.Net, Cancer Forums, and Inspire provide useful materials as well as a sense of community.

9. **Local Support Services:** Many areas have cancer support centers or organizations that provide a variety of services such as transportation, support groups, counseling, and educational programs.

10. **Financial Assistance Programs:** Various organizations and charities aid cancer patients and caregivers with medical bills, transportation fees, and other treatment-related expenditures.

11. **Legal and Advocacy Services:** Some organizations provide legal aid and advocacy services to assist patients and caregivers in navigating insurance, job, and disability benefits concerns.

12. **Wellness Programs:** Cancer wellness programs frequently focus on improving patients' and carers' physical and emotional well-being. Exercise courses, mindfulness training, and dietary counseling may all be part of these programs.

13. **Educational Workshops:** Many cancer clinics and support groups hold educational workshops and seminars to assist patients and caregivers better understand cancer, treatment choices, and coping methods.

14. **Hotlines and Helplines:** Trained experts staff toll-free hotlines and helplines to provide urgent assistance, answer questions, and provide direction.

Navigating a cancer diagnosis and treatment can be difficult, and support options can help significantly. Patients and caregivers are urged to take use of these tools, seek assistance when necessary, and establish a strong support network to improve their physical, emotional, and practical well-being throughout the cancer journey.

Financial considerations related to cancer treatment

Financial issues for cancer treatment are an important part of the cancer experience. Cancer treatment may be expensive, and it's critical for patients and their families to recognize and plan for these financial issues. Here's a rundown of significant financial issues and ways for dealing with them:

1. **Health Insurance:** Carefully review your health insurance policy to ensure that it covers cancer treatment, such as hospital stays, surgeries, chemotherapy, radiation therapy, and prescription medicines.

   - Verify network providers to confirm that your favorite healthcare institutions and experts are covered.

- Understand deductibles, copays, and out-of-pocket maximums. If available, consider purchasing extra insurance.

2. **Treatment expenses:** Depending on the kind and stage of cancer, treatment modes, and length, cancer treatment expenses might vary greatly. Ask your healthcare provider for comprehensive cost estimates.

3. **Treatment Planning:** Discuss treatment alternatives with your healthcare team, keeping the prospective expense of each option in mind. Consider the trade-off between efficacy and cost-effectiveness.

4. **Financial Counseling:** Many hospitals and cancer centers provide financial counseling services to patients to aid them in navigating insurance claims, billing, and financial assistance programs.

5. **Prescription Drug Prices:** Chemotherapy and other treatments can be costly. Inquire with your doctor about cost-effective alternatives, generic prescriptions, and

patient assistance programs provided by drug makers.

6. **Travel and hotel charges:** Depending on the location of your treatment, you may incur travel and hotel charges. Investigate support organizations that aid cancer patients with transportation and lodging.

7. **Employment and Income:** Learn about your employment rights and if you may continue working while undergoing treatment. Some patients may require time off, work fewer hours, or investigate disability benefits.

8. **Disability Benefits:** Investigate your employer's or government programs' short-term and long-term disability benefits. Consult a financial advisor or a legal professional for assistance in obtaining these advantages.

9. **Financial Assistance Programs:** Research financial assistance programs given by government agencies, non-profit groups, and pharmaceutical firms. These programs can

assist with the payment of treatment charges, co-pays, and transportation expenditures.

10. **Budgeting:** Create a budget that accounts for medical bills, everyday living expenses, and future income fluctuations. Prioritize necessary costs while reducing unnecessary spending.

11. **Emergency Fund:** Create an emergency fund or dip into current funds to cover unforeseen medical bills or temporary income loss during treatment.

12. **Legal and Financial Planning:** Review and update legal papers such wills, advance healthcare directives, and powers of attorney. Consult a financial advisor or estate planner for advice on asset management and future planning.

13. **contact:** Maintain open lines of contact with healthcare providers, insurance companies, and billing departments. Correct any billing problems or anomalies as soon as possible.

14. **Seek support:** Don't be afraid to seek support from social workers, financial counselors, or patient advocacy groups that specialize in assisting cancer patients with the financial elements of treatment.

15. Keep careful records of medical spending, insurance claims, and communication with healthcare providers and insurers. This paperwork can be useful for tax purposes as well as for dispute settlement.

Cancer treatment can be emotionally and financially taxing, but smart financial preparation and access to accessible resources can help ease some of the difficulties. Seek the assistance of healthcare specialists and financial consultants to efficiently negotiate the financial implications of cancer treatment. Remember that your health and access to treatment should be your primary priorities throughout your cancer experience.

PROVIDING
EMOTIONAL SUPPORT

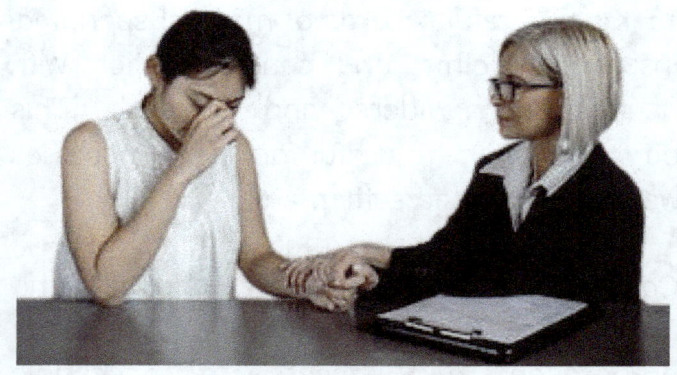

I was told about the story of a lady whose name was *Hilton Sarah*. She was recognized far and wide for her humanitarian personality and unflinching support for people in need. Her life was about to take a turn that would put her remarkable skill of offering emotional support to the test.

One lovely morning, Sarah's friend, Lisa, received a dreadful diagnosis: cancer. The news shocked Lisa's life, leaving her bewildered and afraid. She knew the journey ahead would be tough, both physically and mentally.

Sarah, being the kind person she was, quickly leaped into action. She visited Lisa with a tray of freshly baked muffins and a kind smile that expressed, "I'm here for you." She didn't bombard Lisa with questions or suggestions; instead, she simply listened as Lisa painfully recounted her concerns, disappointments, and anxieties.

Over the ensuing weeks, Sarah became Lisa's constant friend. She drove Lisa to her medical appointments, patiently waiting in the waiting rooms and providing a soothing hand to hold at tough moments. Sarah even investigated the latest therapies and associated side effects, so she could better comprehend what her buddy was going through.

One evening, as they sat on Lisa's porch watching the sunset, Sarah gently broached the idea of support groups. "I've heard that joining a support group can really help cancer patients connect with others who understand their journey," she said. Lisa hesitant at first but finally agreed to give it a try.

Sarah accompanied Lisa to her first support group meeting, where they met other cancer patients and survivors who shared their stories and gave consolation. Lisa was astonished at how much it helped to chat to individuals who could connect to her experiences. She began going frequently, seeking peace and strength in the company of individuals who shared her concerns and hopes.

As Lisa's therapy proceeded, Sarah continued to be her unshakable rock of support. She welcomed every tiny triumph, from completing a round of chemotherapy to regaining her appetite. She also joined in Lisa's moments of sadness, giving a shoulder to weep on and words of encouragement.

One day, Lisa confessed in Sarah that she was trying to come to grips with the changes in her looks due to therapy. Sarah, ever resourceful, linked Lisa with a local group that gave free cosmetic makeovers and wig fits for cancer sufferers. The event gave back a spark of confidence and a grin to Lisa's face.

Over time, Lisa's health began to improve. Her therapies were working, and the cancer was slowly disappearing. Sarah remained by her side, even as the trek got less onerous. Their friendship had developed through shared tears, laughter, and endless cups of tea.

One lovely morning, while Lisa sat in her yard, she turned to Sarah and said, "You've been my rock through all of this. I don't know how I would have coped without you." Sarah smiled, her eyes filling with tears of appreciation. "That's what friends are for," she said quietly.

Their tale serves as a reminder that offering emotional support to a loved one suffering cancer may make an immense impact. Through unshakable friendship and a loving heart, Sarah had helped Lisa discover the fortitude to tackle her obstacles with bravery and optimism.

- Managing caregiver burnout

Managing caregiver burnout is critical for the well-being of persons who offer care and support to loved ones confronting illness, especially cancer. Caregiver burnout can come from the physical, emotional, and mental strain of caregiving over a lengthy period. Here are practical recommendations on how to manage and avoid caregiver burnout:

1. Don't attempt to handle the caring obligations alone. Reach out to family members, friends, and support groups that may give aid and emotional support.

2. Prioritize self-care, which includes obtaining adequate rest, eating a balanced diet, and engaging in regular physical exercise. Caring for yourself helps you to better care for your loved one.

3. Accept that you cannot achieve everything. Set attainable objectives and be compassionate to yourself when you can't

satisfy every requirement. It's alright to ask for aid.

4. Arrange for respite care, which entails temporarily alleviating your caring tasks. This allows you to take a break, regroup, and respond to your own needs.

5. Maintain open communication with your loved one and their healthcare professionals. Discuss your problems, acknowledge your limits, and seek assistance on managing the caregiving position properly.

6. Set clear boundaries to prevent caregiver burnout. Determine your caring limits, explain them to your loved one, and stick to them when required.

7. When friends or relatives volunteer to assist, accept their aid cheerfully. Delegate responsibilities, such as grocery shopping or domestic chores, to ease your workload.

8. Stay socially connected. Isolation may lead to burnout, so make an effort to maintain

your relationships and seek emotional support from friends and loved ones.

9. Organize your caregiving chores efficiently. Create a timetable that provides for breaks and self-care activities while ensuring your loved one's needs are addressed.

10. Consider meeting with a therapist or counselor who specializes in caregiver stress. Therapy can give skills for coping with the emotional issues of caring.

11. Educate yourself on the medical condition your loved one is enduring. Understanding the condition and its course helps alleviate worry and uncertainty.

12. Explore caregiving applications and online tools that can help you organize appointments, prescriptions, and caring duties more effectively.

13. Practice mindfulness practices, such as meditation or deep breathing, to reduce stress and stay grounded during stressful circumstances.

14. Understand that caring can provoke a range of feelings, including guilt, frustration, and despair. Accept these sensations as a typical part of the caring process.

15. Consider long-term planning, including legal and financial arrangements, to guarantee that your loved one's requirements are satisfied in the future.

16. Engage in activities that improve your resilience, such as hobbies, exercise, and spending time with loved ones.

17. Don't disregard your own health. Schedule frequent check-ups with your healthcare practitioner to assess your physical and mental well-being.

Remember that caregiver burnout is widespread, and it's not a show of weakness to seek assistance and prioritize self-care. By applying these measures, carers can lower the risk of burnout and offer better care to their loved ones over the long term.

ASSISTING WITH DAILY LIVING

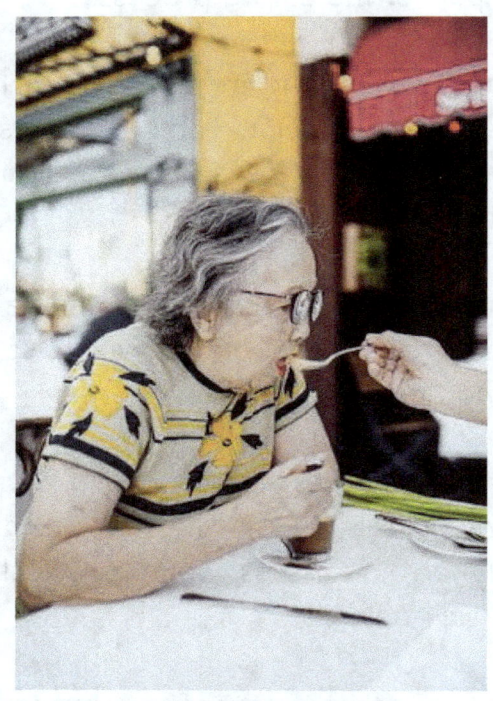

Assisting with everyday functioning is an important element of caregiving for those with cancer or other chronic diseases. It entails offering practical aid and support to ensure that the patient's fundamental requirements are satisfied while retaining their dignity and quality of life. Here are crucial concerns and techniques for aiding with everyday life as a caregiver:

1. Assist the patient with activities of daily living (ADLs), including bathing, dressing, grooming, and toileting, as needed. Be considerate of their privacy and interests.

2. Ensure that the patient takes drugs as recommended. Organize pillboxes, create reminders, and manage medication regimens to prevent missed doses.

3. Provide physical support as necessary for walking, shifting from bed to chair, or utilizing mobility devices such as walkers or wheelchairs.

4. Plan and prepare healthy meals that match with the patient's dietary needs and preferences. Encourage hydration and keep regular meal routines.

5. If the patient has trouble eating themself, aid with feeding while maintaining a pleasant and dignified setting.

6. Help with oral care, including cleaning teeth and denture maintenance, to avoid infections and preserve oral health.

7. If necessary, aid with incontinence care by giving frequent toilet breaks, replacing adult diapers or pads, and maintaining cleanliness.

8. Monitor the patient's skin for any symptoms of pressure sores or skin irritations. Follow physician recommendations for wound care if applicable.

9. Encourage and help with recommended mobility exercises to maintain muscular strength and flexibility. Consult the healthcare staff for guidance.

10. Offer emotional support by actively listening, providing reassurance, and delivering comfort during periods of discomfort or anxiety.

11. Spend meaningful time with the patient engaging in things they love, such as reading, watching movies, or playing games.

12. Ensure a safe atmosphere by eliminating trip hazards, fastening handrails, and installing appropriate safety equipment, including grab bars in the restroom.

13. Foster open dialogue with the patient to understand their requirements, preferences, and concerns. Be patient and sensitive to their verbal and non-verbal clues.

14. Provide transportation to medical appointments, treatments, and other required tasks. Ensure the car is accessible and pleasant for the patient.

15. Be alert in detecting and reporting any adverse drug side effects to the healthcare team.

16. Advocate for the patient's needs within the healthcare system, ensuring they receive adequate treatment and support.

17. If suggested by healthcare experts, help with the use of assistive equipment such as hearing aids, spectacles, or mobility aids.

18. Whenever feasible, encourage the patient to participate in self-care tasks to retain a sense of independence and control.

19. Be flexible and change your caregiving strategy as the patient's requirements and condition vary over time.

20. Don't hesitate to seek assistance from other family members, friends, or respite care services to minimize caregiver burnout and maintain continual support.

Assisting with everyday life involves patience, compassion, and a genuine dedication to the well-being of the patient. Caregivers play a key role in ensuring the patient's comfort, dignity, and overall quality of life during their healthcare journey.

Managing medications and treatments

Managing drugs and therapy is a key job for carers of patients with cancer or chronic diseases. Ensuring that prescriptions are taken appropriately and treatment regimens are followed may substantially improve the patient's well-being and treatment outcomes. Here are crucial tips for efficiently managing drugs and therapy as a caregiver:

1. Medication Organization: Maintain a well-organized system for drugs. Use pillboxes, calendars, or medication management applications to keep track of doses, timetables, and any specific instructions.

2. **Medication record:** Create a detailed record of all the patient's medications, including names, doses, frequencies, and reasons for taking them. Share this list with healthcare providers.

3. **Communication with Healthcare Team:** Maintain open communication with the patient's healthcare team. Keep them updated about any changes in the patient's condition, adverse effects, or concerns regarding drugs or therapy.

4. **Pharmaceutical Labels:** Ensure that pharmaceutical containers are properly labeled with the drug's name, dosing directions, and any risks. Keep all drugs in their original container.

5. **Dosage Accuracy:** Measure liquid drugs accurately using a syringe or measuring cup. Double-check medication doses and deliver them as instructed.

6. **Medicine Reminders:** Set up reminders, alarms, or notifications to prompt medicine administration at the right times. Some cellphones and medication management applications offer this capability.

7. **Adherence to Treatment Plan**: Understand the treatment plan established by the healthcare team, including the timing and duration of drugs and other therapy. Ensure that the patient follows the plan as instructed.

8. **Side Effect Monitoring:** Be careful in monitoring and reporting any side effects or adverse responses to drugs or therapies.

Document these observations for healthcare practitioners.

9. **Special Instructions:** Pay particular attention to special instructions, such as whether prescriptions should be taken with food, on an empty stomach, or at certain intervals.

10. **Medication Storage:** Store drugs correctly, following specified temperature and humidity limits. Keep drugs out of reach of youngsters and dogs.

11. **Refill Management:** Stay ahead of drug refills to avoid pauses in treatment. Consider using mail-order or automated medication refill services for convenience.

12. **Tracking Progress:** Maintain a notebook or record to follow the patient's progress, including symptom changes, improvements, or any concerns connected to therapy.

13. **Consultation with Pharmacists:**
Pharmacists can give essential information regarding drugs, possible interactions, and

adverse effects. Don't hesitate to ask them questions or seek clarification.

14. **Treatment Calendar:** Create a treatment calendar that covers medical appointments, therapy regimens, and drug administration timings. Share this calendar with the patient and healthcare team.

15. **Emergency Medication Kit:** Prepare an emergency medication kit containing vital drugs, medical information, and contact numbers in case of unanticipated occurrences.

16. **Backup Caregiver Plan:** Have a backup plan in place with another trusted caregiver who can step in if you are unable to handle medications and therapy temporarily.

17. **Regular Medication evaluations:** Schedule regular medication evaluations with the healthcare team to appraise the effectiveness of therapy and make any required modifications.

18. **Educate the Patient:** Ensure that the patient knows the necessity of following to their medicine and treatment plan. Encourage them to ask inquiries and voice any concerns.

19. **Safety steps:** Be aware of potential medication-related safety dangers, such as falls or dizziness, and take required steps to prevent accidents.

20. **Seek Professional assistance:** If you find issues in managing drugs and therapy, speak with healthcare experts, including pharmacists and nurses, for assistance and support.

Effective administration of drugs and therapy is vital for the patient's overall health and well-being. Caregivers play a vital role in ensuring that the treatment plan is followed precisely and that any concerns are handled immediately to optimize the patient's chances of recovery or better quality of life.

Nutritional support and meal planning

Nutritional support and meal preparation are key parts of caregiving for those experiencing cancer or other chronic diseases. Proper nutrition has a key part in maintaining the patient's general health, immune system, energy levels, and recuperation. Here are crucial concerns and strategies for providing nutritional support and meal planning as a caregiver:

1. Begin by speaking with the patient's healthcare team, including dietitians or nutritionists, to understand particular dietary requirements and limits depending on the patient's condition, treatment plan, and any side effects.

2. Aim to give a well-balanced diet that contains a range of foods from all dietary categories, such as fruits, vegetables, lean proteins, whole grains, and dairy or dairy substitutes.

3. Encourage the patient to have small, frequent meals and snacks throughout the day, which can help maintain energy levels and minimize nausea or other treatment-related adverse effects.

4. Ensure the patient is appropriately hydrated. Offer water, herbal teas, and clear soups, and check fluid intake, especially if the patient has dehydration due to therapy.

5. Consider the patient's dietary preferences and cultural or religious dietary limitations while arranging meals. Respect their choices while offering healthful options.

6. Many cancer therapies might impair the patient's perception of taste. Adapt meals to accommodate taste changes, such as avoiding strong tastes or textures that may be undesirable.

7. Prioritize nutrient-dense foods that supply important vitamins and minerals. These may include dark leafy greens, berries, lean meats, and whole grains.

8. Ensure the patient eats a proper quantity of protein, since it is vital for tissue regeneration and maintaining muscular mass. Offer lean sources of protein such poultry, fish, beans, and tofu.

9. If the patient has trouble swallowing or chewing due to cancer-related difficulties, try altering the texture of foods to make them simpler to ingest. Puree (a smooth cream of liquidized or crushed fruit or vegetables) or mix meals as needed.

10. Regularly monitor the patient's weight and nutritional status. Report any major weight loss or increase to the healthcare team for examination and modifications to the eating plan.

11. Some patients may require special diets, such as a soft diet or a low-residue diet, based on their individual demands and treatment-related issues. Follow dietary suggestions supplied by healthcare providers.

12. Prepare meals that are easy to digest, appealing in taste and appearance, and

served at suitable temperatures. Include favorite meals wherever feasible.

13. If the patient has nausea, provide bland, non-greasy meals and avoid strong-smelling or spicy foods. Consult with healthcare providers for anti-nausea measures.

14. Discuss the use of nutritional supplements or meal replacement shakes with the healthcare team, as they may be essential to satisfy nutritional requirements.

15. Be conscious of any food allergies or sensitivities the patient may have, and read food labels carefully to avoid potential allergens.

16. Whenever feasible, encourage the patient to participate in meal planning and preparation to retain a sense of freedom and control over their nutrition.

17. Maintain a food journal to document the patient's dietary intake and any adverse responses or food preferences. Share this information with the healthcare staff.

18. Provide emotional support throughout meals, since eating can be emotionally charged for certain patients. Create a peaceful and pleasant dining environment.

19. If you face issues or have questions regarding meal planning and nutrition, don't hesitate to seek help from licensed dietitians or nutritionists.

20. Be flexible with meal planning, since the patient's tastes and nutritional needs may alter over time. Be sensitive to comments and make improvements as appropriate.

Nutritional care and meal planning are crucial to a patient's general well-being and rehabilitation. As a caregiver, your role in delivering nutritional and enticing meals may contribute considerably to the patient's comfort and quality of life during their healthcare journey.

When Patients Refuses Meals Or HealthCare Instructions

Dealing with a patient who refuses to consume meals and follow healthcare recommendations can be tough for caretakers. It's crucial to treat this scenario with kindness, compassion, and tolerance while addressing the underlying causes of their reluctance. Here are measures to consider:

1. Communicate Openly: Initiate a calm and non-confrontational dialogue with the patient to understand their reasons for refusing. Listen carefully and empathetically to their problems, anxieties, or preferences.

2. Respect Autonomy: Respect the patient's autonomy and decision-making capabilities. In other circumstances, people may have solid grounds for their refusal, such as serious side effects from therapy, pain, or personal preferences.

3. Involve the Healthcare Team: Consult the patient's healthcare team to gather insights into the reasons behind the rejection and

discuss possible revisions to the treatment plan or dietary recommendations.

4. Offer alternate alternatives: Propose alternate food alternatives that match with the patient's dietary limitations or preferences. Collaborate with a qualified dietitian or nutritionist to build a more enticing food plan.

5. Address Treatment Side Effects: If the patient's rejection is linked to treatment side effects including nausea, vomiting, or taste changes, discuss these problems with the healthcare team to seek symptom management alternatives.

6. check Vital Signs: Continuously check the patient's vital signs, weight, and overall health. Rapid weight loss or substantial worsening may demand prompt medical attention.

7. Encourage Small, Frequent Meals: Suggest smaller, more frequent meals and snacks throughout the day instead of usual three meals. This technique might be less daunting

for those who have difficulties ingesting greater servings.

8. Include Favorite Foods: Incorporate the patient's favorite foods and comfort items into their meals to make the dining experience more pleasurable and attractive.

9. Create a Pleasant Atmosphere: Ensure that the dining setting is pleasant, free from distractions, and favorable to relaxation. Create a happy and encouraging atmosphere during meals.

10. Offer Support: Offer physical and emotional support during meals, such as sitting with the patient, participating in conversation, and offering mild encouragement without pressure.

11. Educate and Inform: Share information on the significance of nutrition and following healthcare instructions for the patient's well-being and recovery. Sometimes, understanding the rationale helps encourage compliance.

12. Use Visual tools: Visual tools like visual food charts or meal planning diagrams can assist patients better grasp dietary advice and make educated decisions.

13. Seek Professional Guidance: If the patient's rejection persists, consider contacting a psychologist or counselor who specializes in eating disorders, nutrition, or behavioral therapy to address the psychological components of refusal.

14. Consider Tube Feeding: In severe circumstances where the patient's rejection creates a considerable health risk, tube feeding may be explored as a last option. Consult the healthcare team for help on this choice.

15. Document the Refusal: Keep complete records of the patient's refusals, including dates, reasons, and any conversations with the healthcare team. This paperwork can aid in analyzing the patient's progress and decision-making capacity.

16. Monitor Mental Health: Keep an eye on the patient's mental health and emotional well-being. Refusal of meals and healthcare recommendations might be connected to anxiety, sadness, or other psychological disorders that may require treatment.

17. Involve Family and Loved Ones: Engage the patient's family and loved ones to give further support and encouragement. Sometimes, the presence of a familiar person may make a difference.

18. Be Patient and Persistent: Continue to tackle the problem with patience and tenacity. Behavioral adjustments, especially meal acceptance, might take time.

19. Review drugs: Evaluate whether any drugs the patient is taking may be impacting their appetite or taste perception. Discuss suggested modifications with the healthcare team.

20. Legal Considerations: In circumstances where the patient's refusal constitutes a major harm to their health, engage with legal

specialists and healthcare ethics committees to investigate the ethical and legal implications of decision-making.

Remember that refusal of meals and healthcare recommendations might be complex and diverse. The goal is to maintain open communication, address underlying problems, and engage with the healthcare team to identify the most acceptable and compassionate strategy to support the patient's well-being.

MANAGING SIDE EFFECTS

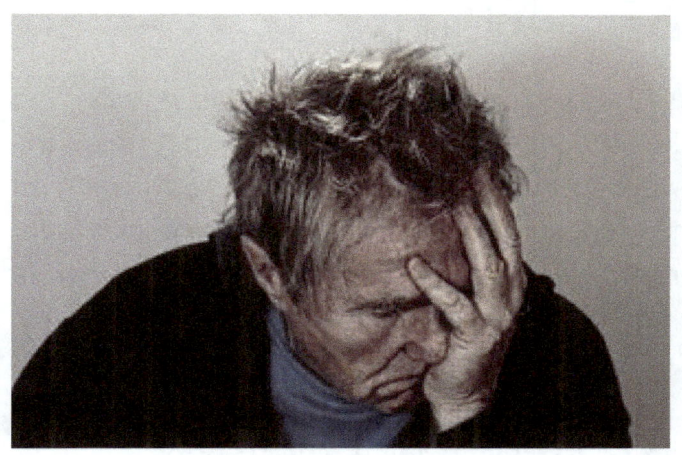

Managing side effects is a key element of caregiving for those battling cancer or through treatment for various medical illnesses. Navigating common side effects such as nausea, exhaustion, and discomfort, working closely with the healthcare team to control symptoms, and reacting to changes in the patient's health are critical components of providing successful treatment. Here's how to tackle these components of caring which has been described earlier in prior sections:

Navigating Common Side Effects:

1. Nausea and Vomiting: Consult with the healthcare team for anti-nausea drugs and ways to ease nausea. Encourage the patient to consume modest, bland meals, and remain hydrated. Ginger and peppermint may also help alleviate nausea.

2. tiredness: Support the patient in managing tiredness by helping them prioritize rest, create a sleep regimen, and engage in light physical exercise as prescribed by the healthcare team. Ensure a comfy sleeping environment.

3. Pain: Work with healthcare providers to address pain management. Administer prescription pain medications on schedule, and urge the patient to describe pain levels properly. Heat or cold treatment, massage,

and relaxation techniques can supplement pain management.

4. Changes in Appetite: - Be adaptive with meal planning to meet variations in the patient's appetite and taste preferences. Encourage smaller, more frequent meals and give nutrient-dense alternatives.

5. Cognitive Changes (Chemo Brain): Recognize and give assistance for cognitive changes, frequently referred to as "chemo brain." Assist the patient with organization, memory aids, and establishing a routine to cope with memory and attention challenges.

Working with the Healthcare Team to Manage Symptoms:

1.Open Communication: Maintain open and transparent communication with the healthcare staff. Report any new or worsening adverse symptoms quickly, since rapid care can frequently avert consequences.

2. Medication Management: Ensure that the patient takes drugs as recommended, especially symptom management meds. Keep a record of drugs, doses, and schedules to prevent mistakes.

3. Follow Healthcare advice: Follow the healthcare team's advice for controlling side effects. This may include dietary adjustments, hydration requirements, physical activity suggestions, or the use of supporting treatments like acupuncture or yoga.

4. Palliative Care and Supportive Services: Discuss palliative care alternatives with the healthcare team to increase the patient's comfort and quality of life. Palliative care focuses on symptom management and emotional support.

Adapting to Changes in the Patient's Health:

1. Regular Assessments: Stay alert in monitoring the patient's health and well-being. Regular examinations by

healthcare providers can assist identify changes in symptoms or treatment efficacy.

2. Adjustment of Care Plan: Be prepared to adjust the caregiving strategy as the patient's health changes. Collaborate with the healthcare team to make appropriate modifications to therapy, symptom management, and daily care routines.

3. Emotional Support: Provide emotional support to the patient at times of physical suffering or symptom exacerbation. Offer reassurance and be attentive to their emotional needs.

4. Decision-Making talks: Engage in talks with the healthcare team and the patient regarding treatment objectives, potential revisions to the treatment plan, and end-of-life care wishes.

5. Advance Care Planning: Consider advance care planning talks, including the development of advance directives and appointing a healthcare proxy, to ensure that

the patient's preferences are honoured in case of substantial health changes.

6. Seek Respite Care: If caring becomes physically or emotionally exhausting due to changes in the patient's condition, consider obtaining respite care or additional help from healthcare professionals or support organizations.

7. Grief and Bereavement Support: Be prepared for the emotional demands of caregiving, especially if the patient's health deteriorates. Seek sorrow and bereavement support services for both the patient and yourself as required.

Remember that controlling side effects and reacting to changes in the patient's health require flexibility, patience, and a solid support network. Collaborating closely with the healthcare team ensures that the patient receives the best possible treatment and symptom management throughout their healthcare journey.

COPING WITH TREATMENT CHANGES AND TRANSITIONS

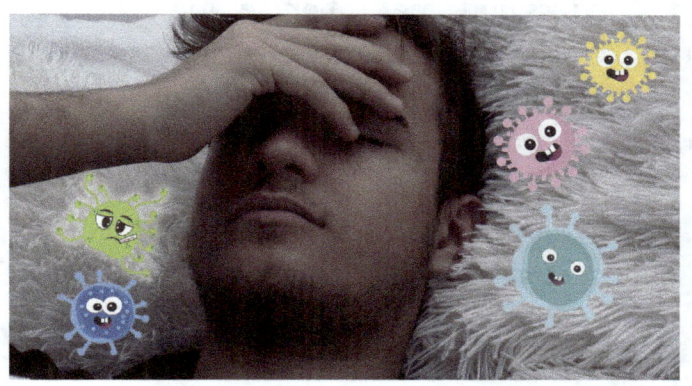

Coping with treatment adjustments and transitions is an important element of caregiving for those battling cancer or chronic diseases. Treatment regimens may alter, and patients may face shifts in their healthcare journey. Here's how to successfully support the patient during these changes:

1. Open Communication: Maintain open and honest communication with the patient.

Discuss any potential therapy adjustments or transitions as early as feasible. Encourage the patient to voice their concerns and desires.

2. Understand the adjustments: Take the time to understand the rationale for treatment adjustments or transitions. Consult with the healthcare team to acquire insights into the medical reasoning and predicted outcomes.

3. Emotional Support: Be attentive to the patient's emotional response to treatment adjustments. They may experience worry, panic, or irritation. Offer emotional support, provide a listening ear, and affirm their sentiments.

4. Seek information regarding the new treatment plan, including potential side effects, duration, and expectations. Knowledge may empower both you and the patient to make educated decisions.

5. Collaborate closely with the healthcare team to facilitate a seamless transition. Ask

inquiries, seek clarification, and get written instructions or care plans if required.

6. Try to maintain a feeling of routine and consistency among treatment changes. Consistency in daily routines, mealtimes, and sleep habits can give comfort.

7. If there are changes in drug regimens, ensure that medicines are changed as per the new treatment plan. Organize prescriptions and set up reminders.

8. Be attentive in monitoring and reporting any new adverse effects or changes in the patient's condition. Early identification can lead to prompt interventions.

9. Consider attending support groups or counseling services for both the patient and yourself to cope with the emotional issues of treatment adjustments.

10. In certain circumstances, it may be advantageous to get a second opinion from another healthcare practitioner, especially if

the patient has concerns about treatment modifications.

11. Advocate for the patient's needs within the healthcare system. Ensure that their preferences and priorities are recognized while making treatment decisions.

12. Practical problems such as transportation to medical visits, insurance coverage, and financial considerations may need to be addressed. Seek aid from social workers or patient advocacy organizations.

13. Be prepared to adjust to changes in the patient's daily life and activities. Modify daily routines as necessary to meet treatment schedules and physical constraints.

14. Encourage the patient to prioritize self-care, including rest, nutrition, and physical exercise to the degree practicable. Caregivers should also exercise self-care to prevent burnout.

15. Keep records of therapy modifications, transition conversations, and any interactions

with the healthcare team. This paperwork can be important for continuity of care.

16. Adjust your expectations and goals in accordance with the new treatment plan. Recognize that certain goals may need to be postponed or changed.

17. Engage in talks regarding the patient's long-term objectives and aspirations for their healthcare journey. This may involve advance care planning and end-of-life care concerns.

18. If coping with treatment changes becomes stressful for either the patient or caregiver, consider obtaining advice from mental health specialists or counselors knowledgeable in healthcare-related concerns.

19. Celebrate treatment milestones, no matter how minor. Recognizing progress may give inspiration and a sense of achievement.

20. Maintain a feeling of hope and optimism throughout the therapy process. Remind the patient that even in the face of changes,

there are often new treatment options and potential for progress.

Coping with treatment adjustments and transitions can be emotionally tough, but with patience, support, and a proactive approach, both caregivers and patients can negotiate these challenges in their healthcare journey with fortitude and drive.

End-of-treatment and survivorship resources

Navigating the completion of treatments and shifting into survivorship is a key milestone in the path of persons who have endured cancer or chronic diseases. It signifies a period of hope, contemplation, and transition to a new era of life. Here's how caregivers may help patients throughout this transition and investigate survival resources:

1. **Celebration and Reflection:** Celebrate the conclusion of therapy as a big success. Take time to reflect on the trip and appreciate the patient's courage and tenacity.

2. **Emotional Support:** Continue to give emotional support throughout this transition phase. The completion of therapy might bring varied feelings, including relief, worry, and uncertainty. Be attention to the patient's feelings and give comfort.

3. **Post-Treatment Assessments:** Attend post-treatment follow-up consultations with the healthcare team as suggested. These assessments assist monitor the patient's development and resolve any lingering problems.

4. **Survivorship Care Plan:** Work with the healthcare team to build a survivorship care plan. This plan contains a timetable for follow-up appointments, necessary testing, and possibly late-term side effect monitoring.

5. **Monitoring Late Effects:** Be careful in monitoring for late-term treatment effects or possible problems. Report any unexpected symptoms to the healthcare staff quickly.

6. **Lifestyle modifications:** Support the patient in making healthy lifestyle modifications

post-treatment. Encourage regular physical exercise, healthy nutrition, and stress management skills.

7. **Psychological help:** Encourage the patient to seek psychological help or therapy if required to address anxiety, depression, or other emotional issues connected to surviving.

8. **Rebuilding Confidence:** Help the patient recover their confidence and self-esteem. Engage in activities that promote a good body image and self-worth.

9. **Return to Normalcy:** Support the patient's efforts to return to a feeling of normalcy in their everyday life. This may entail reestablishing habits, returning to work, or restarting hobbies and interests.

10. **Sexual Health:** Address any problems relating to sexual health or intimacy that may have been compromised by therapy. Encourage open dialogue with healthcare providers.

11. **Financial and Legal problems:** Address any financial or legal problems that may have emerged throughout therapy. Ensure that insurance and legal paperwork are up-to-date.

12. **Support Groups:** Explore survivorship support groups and communities. Connecting with individuals who have gone through similar circumstances may create a sense of belonging and shared insight.

13. **Education and Information:** Continue to educate yourself and the patient on survivorship issues and potential long-term effects of therapy. Knowledge enables informed decision-making.

14. **Late Effect Management:** Be prepared for the possibility of late effects or secondary health issues connected to therapy. Proactive management can lessen the effect of these concerns.

15. **Follow-Up Care:** Ensure that the patient attends planned follow-up appointments and sticks to the survivorship care plan. Regular

check-ins with the healthcare team are vital for maintaining well-being.

16. **Advance Care Planning:** Engage in advance care planning talks. These dialogues can assist the patient explain their healthcare preferences and end-of-life desires.

17. **Wellness Programs:** Explore wellness programs and survivorship-focused initiatives offered by cancer centers, hospitals, and local groups. These may include exercise courses, nutrition workshops, and stress management programs.

18. **Financial Support:** Investigate financial support resources that may be available to survivors, such as grants, scholarships, or financial assistance programs.

19. **Legal Advocacy:** Consider legal advocacy services or groups that specialize in survivorship concerns, including legal matters pertaining to healthcare, employment, and disability.

20. **Celebrate Survivorship:** Celebrate survivorship milestones and anniversaries. Acknowledge the patient's path and resilience. These festivities may serve as strong reminders of strength and optimism.

The shift from treatment to survival is a period of transformation and adjustment. By offering continual support, promoting self-care, and exploring available survivorship options, caregivers may help patients embrace their new chapter with confidence and optimism.

If you liked this, then check out my other book, EATING THAT BEATS DISEASES, the ultimate healthy diet guide to preventing cancer.

END-OF-LIFE CARE

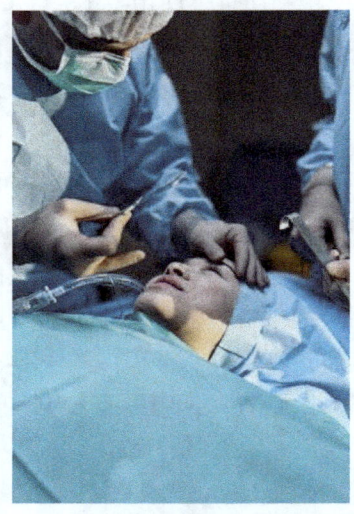

Understanding end-of-life care and planning is a critical element of caregiving, especially for those facing terminal diseases or reaching the end of their lives. This period necessitates a deliberate and caring approach to guarantee the patient's comfort, dignity, and quality of life. Here is a thorough resource on end-of-life care and planning:

- 1. Open and Honest Communication: Initiate open and honest talks with the patient regarding their prognosis and end-of-life desires. Encourage them to voice their desires and concerns about their care.

- 2. Palliative Care vs. Hospice Care: Identify the distinction between palliative care and hospice care. Palliative care focuses on symptom management and enhancing the patient's quality of life, whereas hospice care is for those who have a life expectancy of six months or fewer and offers comfort care.

- 3. Advance Care Planning: Assist the patient in developing advance directives, such as a living will and durable power of attorney for healthcare. These legal agreements define the patient's medical treatment choices and designate a healthcare proxy to make decisions on their behalf if the patient becomes unable to do so.

- 4. Identify Healthcare Proxy: Ensure that the patient's healthcare proxy is identified, informed, and knows their role in making medical choices on the patient's behalf.

- 5. Emotional Support: Offer emotional support to the patient and their family. This is a difficult moment for patients, who may suffer anxiety, sadness, or existential issues. Encourage them to seek out therapy or support groups.

-
- 6. Pain and Symptom Management: Work with the healthcare team to control pain and eliminate uncomfortable symptoms. The patient's comfort is a key goal in end-of-life care.

- 7. Hospice Care Evaluation: If the patient is eligible for hospice care, contact with a hospice service to assess their requirements and decide the best treatment plan. Hospice offers a holistic approach to end-of-life care, including pain treatment, emotional support, and spiritual care.

- 8. Medication Management: Maintain good medication management to ensure that the patient obtains the necessary drugs to address pain, symptoms, and discomfort. Work closely with healthcare providers to modify medicines as required.

- 9. Spiritual and Emotional Needs: Address the patient's spiritual and emotional needs, which may entail contacting religious leaders or spiritual counselors. During this period, patients and families frequently seek spiritual direction and support.

- 10. Comfort Measures: Implement comfort measures such as rotating and repositioning the patient to prevent bedsores, offering mouth care, and maintaining a pleasant and quiet atmosphere.

- 11 Nutrition and Hydration: Discuss and make educated decisions about nutrition and hydration. Some patients may prioritize oral intake, whilst others may prioritize comfort.

- 12. Family Involvement: Include the patient's family in conversations regarding end-of-life care and preparation. Encourage them to communicate their own wants and concerns, and include them in decision-making to the extent that the patient desires.
- 13. Dignity and Respect: Ensure that the patient is treated with dignity and respect throughout his or her end-of-life journey. Consider their cultural, religious, and personal preferences.

- 14. Legacy and Memory-Making: Encourage the patient and family to participate in legacy and memory-making activities. These might involve making memory books, recording messages, or spending quality time together.

- 15. Grief and Bereavement Support: Identify and connect the patient's family with grief and bereavement support services. Bereavement assistance is vital for coping with loss and transitioning to life following the patient's death.

- 16. Legal and Financial Considerations: Address legal and financial issues such as wills, estates, and end-of-life financial preparation. Consult with legal and financial experts as required.

- 17. Funeral and Burial Planning
  - Talk about funeral and burial plans, taking into account the patient's desires as well as religious or cultural norms. Prepare appropriate papers and, if possible, contact funeral services in advance.

- 18. Comfort Care at Home: If the patient prefers to receive end-of-life care at home, ensure that necessary support is available, such as skilled caregivers, medical equipment, and hospice services.

- 19. Time for Closure: Make time for the patient and their loved ones to say their goodbyes, share memories, and achieve closure. This may be a very important and therapeutic experience.

- 20. Be Present: Above all, be present and available to the patient. Your presence, compassion, and company can provide comfort and consolation during this extremely difficult time.

Understanding end-of-life care and planning demands compassion, empathy, and a dedication to following the patient's desires and beliefs. Caregivers may help ensure the patient's final journey is as comfortable and respectful as possible by giving complete support.

CONCLUSION

Your contribution to the patient's journey as a caregiver has been nothing short of outstanding. You've been a rock in their storm, a constant source of support, and the personification of compassion. We've discussed the many obligations and problems you have as a carer throughout this book, from comprehending the intricacies of illness to offering emotional and practical support, from navigating treatments to planning for the future.

Your perseverance, fortitude, and unflinching dedication to your loved one's well-being have blazed a way through even the darkest of times. You've enjoyed victories and survived storms, frequently putting your loved one's demands ahead of your own. Your duty entails more than simply caregiving; it entails love, empathy, and a profound link that surpasses words.

Resources for Ongoing Assistance

Remember that you are never alone on this road of caring. Many resources are available to give guidance, support, and assistance:

- Support Organizations: Joining caregiver support groups, whether in person or online, can put you in touch with people who understand the difficulties you are facing. These communities provide a secure area for people to discuss their experiences, exchange advice, and find consolation in the company of others who are going through similar things.

- Patient Advocacy Groups: Many organizations specialize in providing patients and caregivers with information, services, and advocacy. They can provide advice on the medical, financial, and emotional aspects of caregiving.

- Palliative and Hospice Care Services: Hospice and palliative care programs offer specialist assistance for both patients and carers during end-of-life care. They concentrate on symptom control, comfort, and emotional well-being.

- Psychological Services: Seeking the advice of mental health specialists, such as therapists or counselors, may help you deal with the emotional problems of caring while also maintaining your own mental health.

- Supplemental Care: Don't be afraid to look into respite care services, which may provide carers with short reprieve. Taking pauses and looking after yourself is critical to maintaining your capacity to care for your loved one.

- Resources from the Local Community: To assist you in your caring duty, your local community may provide resources such as meal delivery services, transportation assistance, and home health aides.

- Legal and Financial Consultants: If you're dealing with complicated legal or financial difficulties, consider talking with specialists who specialize in healthcare and caring.

Credits and acknowledgements

Many individuals and organizations worked together to make this book possible. We would like to express our deepest appreciation to:

- The patients and caregivers who kindly offered their ideas and experiences, paving the route for others on this journey.

- The healthcare professionals who work relentlessly to provide excellent treatment, counseling, and support to patients and families.

- Advocacy and support organizations that provide important information and foster communities of understanding.

- Our friends and family who never wavered in their love, encouragement, and support.

- The authors, researchers, and healthcare specialists whose skills and knowledge contributed to the book's content.

- The publishers, editors, and designers who turned words into valuable resources.

Most importantly, thank you for your unending love and devotion as a caretaker. You are the unsung hero in this narrative, and your importance cannot be overstated.

As you continue on your caring path, may you find comfort in knowing that you are making a significant impact in your loved one's life. May you also remember to take care of yourself, to seek help when you need it, and to treasure the moments of connection and love that make the trip worthwhile.

With heartfelt gratitude,

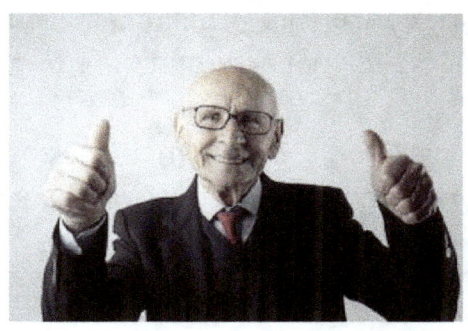

Appendix

List of resources for patients and caregivers

The following materials and tools can be beneficial to patients and caregivers:

1. **American Cancer Society:**
   -[www.cancer.org] (https://www.cancer.org/) The American Cancer Society provides comprehensive cancer information, treatment choices, support services, and caregiver resources.

2. **National Cancer Institute:**
   -[www.cancer.gov] (https://www.cancer.gov/) The National Cancer Institute (NCI) provides thorough cancer information, clinical trials, and support for patients and caregivers.

3. **CancerCare:** Visit their website at [www.cancercare.org].(https://www.cancercare.org/)

CancerCare provides patients and caregivers with counseling, support groups, financial aid, and educational resources.

4. CAN (Caregiver Action Network):
 - http://www.caregiveraction.org/
 - CAN supports caregivers with support, education, and resources.

5. National Alliance for Caregiver Support:
URL:www.caregiving.org
This group provides caregivers with research, advocacy, and support.

6. American Cancer Society (AACR):
 [www.aacr.org] (https://www.aacr.org/)
The American Association for Cancer Research (AACR) provides information about cancer research, clinical trials, and patient resources.

7.Cancer Support Community:
www.cancersupportcommunity.org

For patients and caregivers, this organization provides support groups, education, and wellness activities.

8. National Family Caregivers Association (NFCA):

www.thefamilycaregiver.org](https://www.thefa milycaregiver.org/)

- The NFCA offers services and assistance to family caregivers.

9. Medicare:

Web-Address:[www.medicare.gov](https://www. medicare.gov/)

This official website gives information about healthcare coverage and benefits if the patient is qualified for Medicare.

10. Patient Advocacy Foundations:

Organizations such as the Patient Advocate Foundation (PAF) offer aid with insurance, access to treatment, and financial issues.

http://www.patientadvocate.org/(https://www.p atientadvocate.org/)

11. **Cancer-particular Organizations:**
Depending on the kind of cancer, there are particular organizations that offer disease-specific information, such as the Leukemia & Lymphoma Society, American Lung Association, and Susan G. Komen.

12. **Support Groups and Online Communities:**
Websites such as Inspire, Cancer Survivors Network, and Smart Patients enable patients and caregivers to connect, share stories, and seek guidance.

13. **Caregiving Apps:** Apps such as CaringBridge, Lotsa Helping Hands, and CareZone can help carers organize care duties, manage prescriptions, and communicate with friends and family.

Keep in mind that the particular materials required will vary depending on the patient's diagnosis, treatment plan, and personal circumstances. It is best to get individualized advice and recommendations from healthcare experts, social workers, and patient advocacy organizations.

MEDICATION TRACKERS

MEDICATION TRACKER

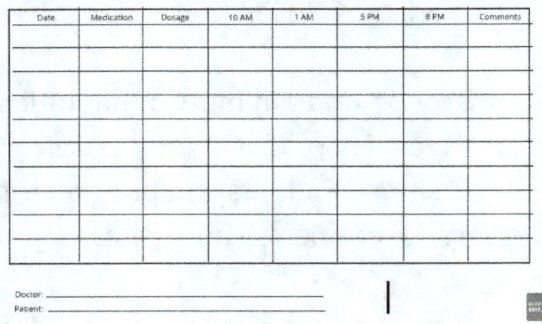

Date	Medication	Dosage	10 AM	1 AM	5 PM	8 PM	Comments

Doctor: _____
Patient: _____

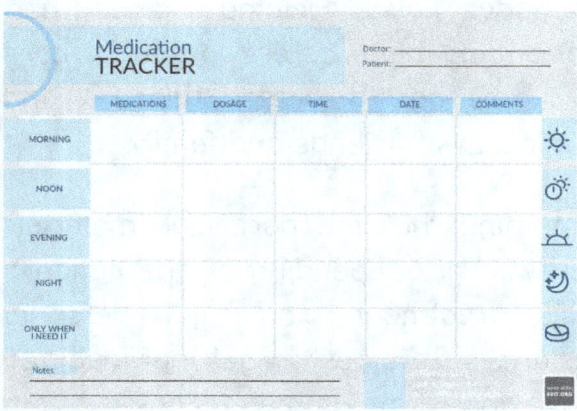

Medication TRACKER

Doctor: _____
Patient: _____

	MEDICATIONS	DOSAGE	TIME	DATE	COMMENTS	
MORNING						
NOON						
EVENING						
NIGHT						
ONLY WHEN I NEED IT						

Notes: _____

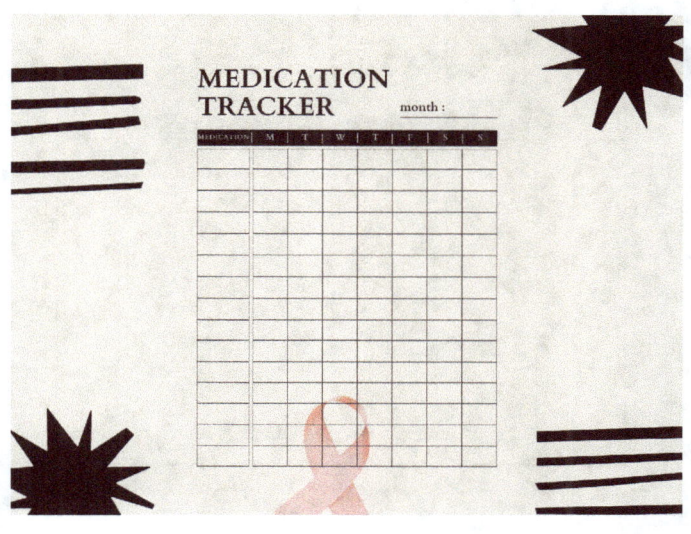

MEDICATION TRACKER   MONTH:_____

#	MEDICATION NAME	1	2	3	4	5	6	7	8	9	10	11	12	13	14	15	16	17	18	19	20	21	22	23	24	25	26	27	28	29	30	31
1																																
2																																
3																																
4																																
5																																
6																																
7																																
8																																
9																																
10																																
11																																
12																																
13																																
14																																
15																																

NOTES

MEDICAL APPOINTMENT TRACKER

DATE	DOCTOR /PROVIDER	PURPOSE OF VISIT	LOCATION	APPOINTMENT STATUS	FOLLOW-UP NOTES

Monthly Medication Tracker

JAN   FEB   MAR   APR   MAY   JUNE   JULY   AUG   SEPT   OCT   NOV   DEC

HABIT	1	2	3	4	5	6	7	8	9	10	11	12	13	14	15	16	17	18	19	20	21	22	23	24	25	26	27	28	29	30	31

Notes

Goals

2023	Monday	Tuesday	Wednesday	Thursday	Friday	Saturday	Sunday	Monday	Tuesday	Wednesday	Thursday
01 JANUARY							1	2	3	4	5
02 FEBRUARY		1	2	3	4	5	6	7	8	9	
03 MARCH			1	2	3	4	5	6	7	8	9
04 APRIL						1	2	3	4	5	6
05 MAY	1	2	3	4	5	6	7	8	9	10	11
06 JUNE				1	2	3	4	5	6	7	8
07 JULY						1	2	3	4	5	6
08 AUGUST	1	2	3	4	5	6	7	8	9	10	
09 SEPTEMBER				1	2	3	4	5	6	7	
10 OCTOBER						1	2	3	4	5	6
11 NOVEMBER		1	2	3	4	5	6	7	8	9	
12 DECEMBER					1	2	3	4	5	6	7

MONTHLY MEDICATION TRACKER

MONTH:		WEEK OF:							
#	MEDICATION	M	T	W	T	F	S	S	
1									
2									
3									
4									
5									
6									
7									
8									
9									
10									

MONTH:		WEEK OF:							
#	MEDICATION	M	T	W	T	F	S	S	
1									
2									
3									
4									
5									
6									
7									
8									
9									
10									

MONTH:		WEEK OF:							
#	MEDICATION	M	T	W	T	F	S	S	
1									
2									
3									
4									
5									
6									
7									
8									
9									
10									

MONTH:		WEEK OF:							
#	MEDICATION	M	T	W	T	F	S	S	
1									
2									
3									
4									
5									
6									
7									
8									
9									
10									

MEDICATION
+ TRACKER

MONTH: _____

_____	○	○	○	○	○	○	○	○	○	○	○	○	○
_____	○	○	○	○	○	○	○	○	○	○	○	○	○
_____	○	○	○	○	○	○	○	○	○	○	○	○	○
_____	○	○	○	○	○	○	○	○	○	○	○	○	○
_____	○	○	○	○	○	○	○	○	○	○	○	○	○
_____	○	○	○	○	○	○	○	○	○	○	○	○	○

MEDICATION SCHEDULE
MONTH OF

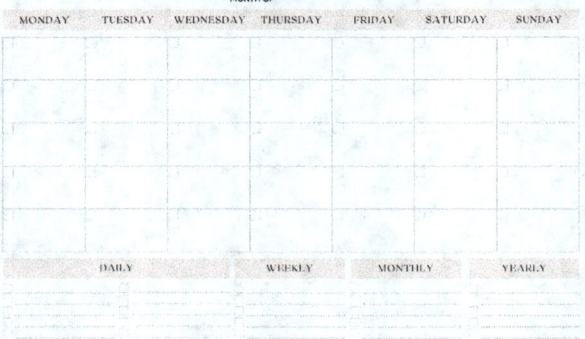

MONDAY	TUESDAY	WEDNESDAY	THURSDAY	FRIDAY	SATURDAY	SUNDAY

DAILY	WEEKLY	MONTHLY	YEARLY

Feel free to enlarge and duplicate